Actinic Keratosis

Replace uncertainty with knowledge: how to prevent recurrence and lower your skin cancer risk

Explains Actinic Keratosis, Solar or Senile Keratosis and Squamous Cell Carcinoma including symptoms and treatments

By

Anthony Newton

Published by Adhurst Publishing Ltd. 2014

Table of Contents

Introduction

A diagnosis of actinic keratosis stimulates a range of emotions and a multitude of questions. How dangerous is this? Am I going to get skin cancer? Why did this happen? Is there anything I can do to help myself?

No book is a good substitute for quality medical care. However, even the best of doctors is hurried, overbooked and sometimes unmindful of the fact that their patients don't have the assurance that comes with a medical education. Even a caring physician can be so focused on treatment of the condition that they forget to treat the emotions and concerns that come with it.

The most unsettling things about a diagnosis of actinic keratosis are the uncertainty, fear and helplessness that you feel, even after treatment. The purpose of this book is to replace uncertainty with knowledge, fear with reassurance and helplessness with positive action.

Within the pages of this book, you'll learn what you need to know about actinic keratosis in its various forms, what treatments are available and what's involved in those treatments, what risk factors led to your actinic keratosis and also what changes you can make and steps you can take to prevent a recurrence and lower your risk of developing skin cancer.

We'll also discuss the emotional aspect of being diagnosed with actinic keratosis – both what you can expect and what you can do to deal with the array of emotions that a diagnosis can bring.

A diagnosis of actinic keratosis is scary. But you do not have to deal with it unarmed. This book will give you the tools you need to take charge of your health and get back to living a full and active life.

Chapter 1 - What is Actinic Keratosis?

When you're diagnosed with any potentially dangerous condition, you immediately have a number of questions, all of which you would prefer to have answered immediately. Many of these questions don't even occur to you until you've left the doctor's office. Unanswered questions, particularly those that start with "why," are a breeding ground for anxiety and fear. One of the main goals of this book is to reduce some of that stress.

In this chapter, we'll discuss what actinic keratosis is, the most common causes of actinic keratosis and which factors put you at risk of developing it.

Actinic Keratosis - The Most Common Precancerous Lesion

When you receive a diagnosis of any condition, the first thing you want and need to know is what you're dealing with.

Most people newly diagnosed with actinic keratosis or anything else find that they have more questions after they *leave* the doctor's office than they did when they went *in*. This is perfectly normal and it's unrealistic to expect your doctor to anticipate and answer every question that may pop into your mind long after your appointment.

In this chapter, you'll learn the basics of what actinic keratosis is, what it looks like, what causes it and what you can expect in the way of a prognosis.

Most people diagnosed with actinic keratosis had never heard of the condition before they found themselves facing it. However, actinic keratosis is actually the most commonly diagnosed "pre-cancerous" skin lesion. We say "pre-cancerous" because while actinic keratosis can lead to squamous cell carcinoma or some other form of skin cancer, skin cancer is not a forgone conclusion. (It's important for you to

10

remember that skin cancer is a real possibility if you've been diagnosed with actinic keratosis, but it is still only a *possibility*.)

According to the American Skin Cancer Foundation, 58 million Americans are diagnosed with actinic keratosis each year (Actinic Keratosis 2013). The UK's Primary Care Dermatology Society reports that 23% of people over 60 in the UK have some form of actinic keratosis, although there are many more cases in patients ranging from ages 30-60 (Actinic keratosis 2011). Incidence is very high in sunny climates and those close to the Equator, with places like Australia ranking high on the list of areas where actinic keratosis is most often diagnosed.

Considering that actinic keratosis is the most commonly diagnosed precancerous lesion, it's safe to assume that there are huge numbers of people who have actinic keratosis but haven't seen a doctor or been diagnosed. Many people with smaller or less severe lesions simply assume that they are warts or some other minor skin problem that will go away on their own. This is one of the most troubling problems with actinic keratosis, as early detection is the most important factor in a good outcome.

The Causes of Actinic Keratosis

Actinic keratosis is directly related to UV damage, either from the sun itself or from exposure to UV rays through tanning beds, tanning lamps and other sources. In general, it's thought that the more prolonged the exposure to UV rays and the more damage done to the skin, the more likely it is that a person will eventually have some form of actinic keratosis. However, it's important to remember that just one sunburn can cause enough damage to stimulate melanoma, the deadliest form of skin cancer. It's safe to say that the same is true of actinic keratosis. While your risk goes up with each exposure to the sun, any exposure can effectively lead to actinic keratosis.

However, statistics point to actinic keratosis being a result of cumulative damage or repeated exposure to the sun and other sources of UV rays.

Who is at Greatest Risk?

Exposure to the sun is the main factor, but not the only risk factor in developing actinic keratosis.

Gender: Men are more likely to develop actinic keratosis than are women. There are a couple of possible reasons for this. First, women are statistically more likely to use some form of skin protection when they are outdoors, such as sunblock or a hat. In fact, most women apply at least some degree of sun protection when they put on their make-up, as most foundations and moisturizers today contain at least some sunscreen. Second, there are generally more men whose work takes them outdoors than there are women. Occupations such as construction, road work, landscaping, roofing and so on are traditionally held by more men than women and all involve spending hours outdoors each day.

Ethnicity: As with melanoma and other forms of skin cancer, you're far more likely to develop actinic keratosis if you are fair-skinned and have light-colored eyes and hair. People with red hair are at the greatest risk, as most of them also have freckles and very fair skin that burns easily. People of Scandinavian descent, with light hair, eyes and skin, are also at a higher risk than many other ethnicities. Actinic keratosis is very rare in people of Asian and African heritage.

The reason for this is the amount of melanin in the skin. Melanin is a naturally-occurring compound in the skin created by cells called melanocytes. The purpose of melanin is to give your skin, eyes and hair their color. The more melanin present in your body, the darker your eyes, skin and hair. By the same token, people who have less melanin in their bodies have lighter skin, blue or green eyes and shades of blonde, red or very light brown hair. It's all about your genetics (Habif, TP 2009).

But melanin is not just a decorative substance – it's also a protective one. UV rays, from the sun or any other source, damage and can destroy the cells of your skin, starting with the topmost layer, the epidermis. Prolonged exposure will cause that damage to penetrate more deeply through the seven layers of skin, from the dermis to the hypodermis.

Sun damage is a burn like any other. We classify burns as either first, second or third-degree burns. First degree burns affect the topmost layer (the epidermis) of the skin and third-degree burns have penetrated to the innermost layer of the skin, the hypodermis. Sunburns are categorized in the same way and even mild sunburn is considered a first-degree burn.

Tanning is actually an *immune* response to the damage caused by the sun and other UV rays.

When the first signs of damage from UV rays are detected in the skin (often within minutes of exposure), melanin is sent to the site to heal and protect the skin cells affected. This is why those people with more melanin in their skin tan so quickly; they have plenty of melanin in their body to race to the skin's surface. This is also why those people with little melanin burn so quickly; they simply don't have enough melanin in their skin to protect them.

Many people make the mistake of believing that if they tan fairly easily, it's safer for them to expose themselves to the sun's damaging rays. But a tan is itself evidence of skin damage; these people are just able to be somewhat protected from more severe damage longer than those who burn more easily.

Age: Actinic keratosis is considered a cumulative disorder. In other words, it's usually a result of repeated or prolonged sun damage. For this reason, it's very common in people over 45 and becomes more common as we age. In fact, some research indicates that virtually everyone over the age of 80 will have at least one actinic keratosis and usually several. (Actinic Keratosis 2013)

While it stands to reason that you're at greater risk for developing actinic keratosis if you're over 40, actinic keratosis has been diagnosed in much younger people who have had a good deal of exposure to the sun. Younger people who spend a good deal of time participating in outdoor sports such as skiing, surfing, running, hiking, sailing and climbing account for many of the younger patients diagnosed with actinic keratosis. Frequent sunbathing is also a common cause for diagnosis at a younger age.

Essentially, you are more likely to develop actinic keratosis in your forties and beyond, but if you do spend a good amount of time in the sun and/or you have had several sunburns, you can find yourself facing actinic keratosis at a much younger age.

Geography: Geography is not as great a risk factor as the others we've just discussed, but it does figure into the statistics. The sun is strongest at the equator, so people in countries like Ecuador are at greater risk, geographically, than those living in France.

Also, people living in a temperate climate tend to spend more time outdoors, so if you're fair-skinned and live in an area where it's warm and sunny most of the year, like Florida, you're potentially at greater risk than someone who is equally fair-skinned but lives in Vermont. However, the time you actually spend out in the sun and whether you use skin protection have a great deal to do with that risk, much more so than where you live.

Immune Health: As we've said, tanning is a result of melanin's role in the immune response to sun exposure. While the genetic factors determining the amount of melanin in your body impact this response, a compromised immune system can as well. Several studies have shown that people with compromised immunity due to chemotherapy, organ transplantation or even excessive UV exposure are also at a higher risk of developing actinic keratosis. It serves to reason, then, that poor immune health on a less dramatic scale can also inhibit your body's ability to protect your skin. (Later in the book, we'll discuss several very effective ways to boost your immune health and help prevent a recurrence of actinic keratosis.)

One of these risk factors may apply to you or several of them may be applicable. There are some risk factors that are out of your control, such as your gender and genetics. However, there are lifestyle and health factors that are somewhat under your control and that you can change or improve from this point forward. It's important for you to know that you are not a hapless or helpless victim to actinic keratosis. There are things you can do to improve your long-term prognosis and, as you're about to read, the prognosis for actinic keratosis is generally good if caught early on.

The Prognosis for Actinic Keratosis

Although having a skin lesion diagnosed as "precancerous" is alarming, you can take some reassurance from the fact that *most* actinic keratoses do *not* progress to skin cancer. They can do so and they do indicate a predisposition for developing some form of skin cancer, but in general the prognosis for most people is very good.

In a recent study published in the *Journal of the American Academy of Dermatology*, it was reported that the incidence of actinic keratosis progressing to skin cancer is actually fairly low.

Five clinical research studies were reviewed that covered a period from 1988 to 1998. Published risk of progression of actinic keratoses to invasive squamous cell carcinoma for individual lesions ranged from 0.025% to

16% per year. Extrapolation from these clinical studies suggests a rate of risk of progression of actinic keratoses to invasive squamous cell carcinoma of approximately 8% taken as an average among the cited statistical rates in the studies reviewed. (RG 2000)

Another study published by Australian researchers was conducted over a period of five years. The study included 1,689 people aged forty or older who had at least one actinic keratosis. At the first examination, the total number of actinic keratoses was 21,905.

All told, there were 4,267 examinations of these patients (for the entire group) during the course of the study. The results from this study were also very encouraging.

A squamous cell carcinoma (SCC) developed within 12 months on 28 of the 4,267 occasions. Where accurate mapping of both SCCs and pre-existing solar keratoses was available, it was found that 10/17 (60%) SCCs arose from a lesion diagnosed clinically as a solar keratosis in the previous year and the other 7 (40%) SCCs on what had been clinically normal skin 12 months previously. The risk of malignant transformation of a solar keratosis to SCC within 1 year was less than 1/1000. (Marks R; Rennie G; Selwood TS 1988)

These are excellent numbers by any standard, but if you're one of the people who have been diagnosed with at least one actinic keratosis, you may not feel as comfortable with the odds as the casual reader would be. That's perfectly natural, as fear has a tendency to overwhelm mathematics.

However, you should focus on those numbers as a very real and scientifically sound indication that most people do not eventually develop skin cancer and the statistics point to you being one of "most people." Later on in this book, we'll discuss some ways you can increase your chances of having an excellent outcome.

There are a few things that influence the probability that someone with actinic keratosis will develop squamous cell carcinoma (the form of skin cancer associated with actinic keratosis).

Number of Lesions: The more lesions a patient has, the more likely they are to have at least one of those lesions develop into squamous cell carcinoma. There's some debate about the reason for this. It may be simple mathematics – the more lesions you have, the more likely that one of them will progress. Or it may be that people with a significant number of actinic keratoses are more predisposed to developing squamous cell carcinoma.

However, some studies have found that people with ten or more lesions are more likely to develop skin cancer at some point. According to the UK's Primary Care Dermatology Society, people with ten or more lesions have a 14% chance of developing squamous cell carcinoma within five years (Actinic keratosis 2011). For this reason, the main objective of treatment is to keep the number of lesions at any one time to a minimum. The fact is that once you have an actinic keratosis, the statistics say you'll continue to get them. Keeping them to a minimum will reduce your risk that one of them will become cancerous. (Actinic Keratosis 2013)

Early Detection: As with skin cancer, early detection and diagnosis is the key. Although the statistics on the prognosis for actinic keratosis are good, there is still a very real danger that one lesion can turn into squamous cell carcinoma. A 2012 study published in the *American Journal of the Academy of Dermatology* put it very simply and very well:

Although most individual ACTINIC KERATOSIS lesions do not become invasive cancers, the majority of invasive squamous cell carcinomas originate from ACTINIC KERATOSIS. (Rigel DS, Stein Gold LF 2013)

Early detection can be a problem for those who haven't already been diagnosed with an actinic keratosis. As you'll read in the next section, many lesions can be small and look fairly innocent. They may be scratched off and then reappear a few months later. Many lesions look much like warts. It's easy to overlook many actinic keratoses or to assume that they're not anything important enough to require a visit to the doctor.

Once you've had an actinic keratosis, though, you'll learn to spot problems early on, to tell the difference (in most cases) between an actinic keratosis and some other benign skin lesion, and you'll likely be getting regular skin examinations from your doctor as well. This will make early detection as likely as it is essential.

Self-care: One of the biggest influences on your prognosis with actinic keratosis will be how you take care of your skin and your general health after treatment. We'll go into self-care in greater detail later on, but once you've had an actinic keratosis, it is essential to protect your skin from further sun damage to prevent or reduce the number of actinic keratoses in the future. This, in turn, will lower your risk of developing squamous cell carcinoma. Boosting your immunity is another way to reduce your risk and we'll talk about that in great detail in the next section.

However, early detection and treatment remain the very best preventive measure and knowing what to look for when examining your own skin is the key to getting treatment as quickly as possible.

Chapter 2 – Recognizing and Diagnosing Actinic Keratosis

The early detection of actinic keratosis is the single most important factor in a healthy outcome. Your doctor will diagnose your lesion, but from then on you'll need to be able to carefully watch your own skin and recognize any new lesions as early as possible.

In this chapter, we'll explain how to identify an actinic keratosis and also what to expect during your appointments for both your first exam and any subsequent examinations.

Recognizing Actinic Keratosis

A thorough examination by your primary care physician or dermatologist is the only way to correctly diagnose or rule out actinic keratosis. However, once you have had actinic keratosis, you are almost certainly going to continue to see new lesions, especially as you age. As with skin cancer and breast cancer, regular self-examination of your skin at home is the key to quickly spotting any changes that may indicate a problem. You need to know where to expect new lesions and how to spot them in their earliest stages.

There is no one "typical" actinic keratosis. The color, size, shape and texture of an actinic keratosis can vary widely from one person to another and even from one lesion to another on the same individual. Much of this has to do with how old the lesion is and how far it's progressed. However, there are several characteristics to look for. Once you've familiarized yourself with them, you'll be better equipped to notice a possible problem very quickly.

Where to Look

Typically, actinic keratoses are found on the parts of the body that are exposed most often to the sun and for longer periods of time. These include the face, ears, scalp, back of the neck, upper chest, forearms, hands and feet but any area that has been exposed to the sun is at risk, especially if there has been significant or repeated sunburn to the area.

What to Look For

While the color, shape and surface of an actinic keratosis will vary, there are certain characteristics common to actinic keratosis.

Most lesions are less than 0.5cm in diameter and they rarely get larger than 1cm in diameter. That can make them a bit easy for you to miss, especially if they're in an area that you can't see very well, such as on your scalp or the top of your ear.

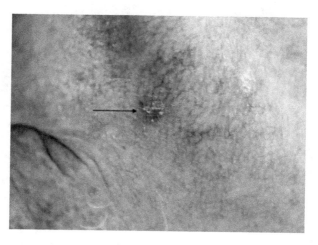

Image courtesy of The Primary Care Dermatology Society (PCDS)

This lesion would be hard to detect during a self-exam unless you knew what to look for.

Lesions can be one or more of several colors. The most typical are white, pink, red, grayish or very close to your skin color.

Actinic keratoses usually start out fairly flat and somewhat shiny, but soon develop a rough or scaly surface. In the beginning, it may be easier to feel that rough surface than it is to see it. Later on, that scaly surface can be an entirely different color than with the original lesion.

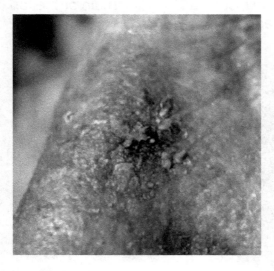

Image courtesy of The Primary Care Dermatology Society (PCDS)

An example of rough, scaly actinic keratosis on the nose.

Very often, you'll notice a lesion that is partly white or skin-colored and partly brown or gray. That inconsistency in color is one of the "red flags" for most types of skin cancer and for actinic keratosis as well. It signifies change and change is not generally considered a good thing.

A variance in the surface of the lesion is another red flag. If part of the surface is smooth and another area becomes scaly, rough, bumpy or thicker than the rest, this is a sign that it may be an actinic keratosis and should be seen by a doctor immediately.

Many lesions take a wart-like appearance and are often mistaken for warts.

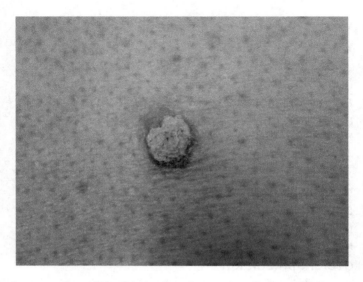

Image courtesy of The Primary Care Dermatology Society (PCDS)

Example of a fairly common type of actinic keratosis. Note the similarity to a common wart.

Some other things to watch out for are any lesions that itch, begin to bleed or that return after being scratched off or shaved accidentally.

In some cases, a small, horn shaped lesion may develop; typically skin colored. These are called cutaneous horns and should be seen by a doctor right away, as they may be a sign that the actinic keratosis has progressed to squamous cell carcinoma.

30

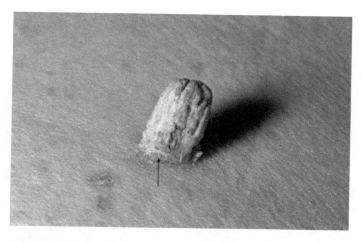

Image courtesy of The Primary Care Dermatology Society (PCDS)

Example of a cutaneous horn. These can appear anywhere but are quite common on the face and ears.

The most important thing to watch for is change. Any kind of change in a lesion is suspect and might include:

- A change in allover color or a lesion that has more than one color.
- A change in the surface of a lesion – the lesion may become raised or scaly.
- A change in the size of the lesion.
- A lesion that goes away or is accidentally scratched or shaved off and then returns.

- Increased or new redness surrounding the lesion.
- New itchiness or pain upon touch.

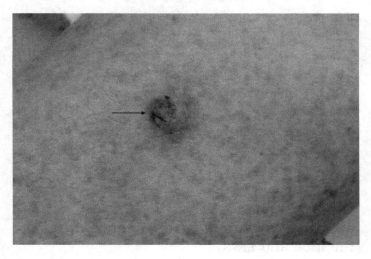

Image courtesy of The Primary Care Dermatology Society (PCDS)

An example of squamous cell carcinoma. Note the presence of two different colors in the lesion.

These are all things that you need to keep in mind when examining your own skin. For areas that you can't easily examine yourself, such as the scalp or back of the neck, it's helpful to have a spouse, relative or friend who can check those areas for you regularly.

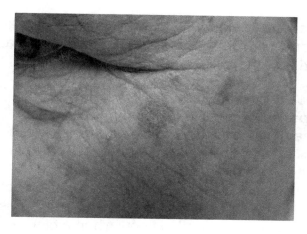

Image courtesy of The Primary Care Dermatology Society (PCDS)

Some lesions are easy to mistake for age or sun spots, but will be scaly or rough in texture, rather than smooth.

If you see anything that meets some of these criteria, you should schedule an appointment with your doctor immediately.

How Actinic Keratosis is Diagnosed

Most instances of actinic keratosis can be fairly accurately diagnosed by clinical examination.

If you first visit your primary care physician, he or she may feel comfortable diagnosing and treating the lesion themself or may choose to refer you to a dermatologist for a thorough skin examination, any biopsies that may be needed and both the initial and ongoing treatment.

Because actinic keratosis is very common, especially in people over forty, your primary care physician can probably recognize these lesions. However, a dermatologist is often a better choice for removal and ongoing treatment. Also, a dermatologist is usually better able to distinguish between the different types of actinic keratosis and to know when a biopsy is called for. They also may have more removal options readily at hand than a primary care physician.

The Examination

Whether your first visit is to your primary care physician or a dermatologist, an examination of the lesion or lesions is the first step to diagnosing it properly.

Your doctor will probably ask several questions such as when you noticed the lesion, if there have been any changes in it since you noticed it and whether you spend a good deal of time out in the sun. Then the doctor will examine the lesion and the skin surrounding it. Typically,

34

actinic keratosis will appear in an area where other signs of sun damage are present, such as wrinkling, sun spots, red or brown discoloration or uneven pigmentation of the skin and so on.

There are certain characteristics of actinic keratosis that your doctor will look for, often by touching and manipulating the area as much as examining it visually. Your doctor will be checking the texture or surface of the lesion and the texture of the skin beneath and surrounding the lesion.

There are several sub-types of actinic keratosis. For the most part, these are descriptive names that detail the location and appearance of the actinic keratosis, rather than differentiating or categorizing the severity of the lesion.

Bowenoid actinic keratosis – also known as Bowen's disease, Bowenoid actinic keratosis is the exception to the above rule. Bowenoid actinic keratosis is actually the earliest stage of squamous cell carcinoma. (James C, Crawford R, Martika M. Actinic Keratosis. In: C. James, R. Crawford, M. Martinka, and R. Marks. 2006)

Although it typically is quite scaly and rough in appearance, many other types of actinic keratosis are also quite scaly, so don't be alarmed if this sounds like *your* lesion. Only a biopsy can definitively diagnose Bowenoid actinic keratosis.

Lichenoid actinic keratosis – Lichenoid actinic keratosis is typically a single lesion, often almost perfectly round and typically red or pink in color.

It's often mistaken for or initially appears to be a regressed lesion. In other words, it often appears at first to be the scar or mark left behind after a planar wart (a small, flat wart often found on the feet) or dysplastic nevus (a benign mole that has gone through changes) has disappeared or been removed. It's no more harmful than any other actinic keratosis. Lichenoid actinic keratosis is simply a descriptive term.

Hypertrophic actinic keratosis – Hypertrophy can most simply be defined as rapid cell building. It's most often used when talking about building new muscle tissue.

A hypertrophic actinic keratosis is typically a rather thick lesion, though most of that thickness may be below the skin's surface. A physician may feel it by palpating the area. Again, the name simply describes the appearance of the lesion, although due to the thickness of a hypertrophic lesion and its below-surface growth, cryotherapy and other non-invasive treatments such as chemical peeling are usually not applicable. Typically, curettage (cutting away the lesion) is the only effective method of removal.

Hyperkeratotic actinic keratosis –
hyperkeratotic actinic keratosis is indicated by a thick scaly crust on the skin and can show as a hornlike protrusion of tissue above the skin. While it can be quite scary looking, it is no more dangerous than any other form of actinic keratosis, though your doctor may want to check there is not a more serious lesion beneath the scaly surface.

Some physicians may opt to use curettage to remove the lesion, but cryotherapy is also a viable choice. If your doctor diagnoses hyperkeratotic actinic keratosis, discuss all of your treatment options with him before deciding which route is the best.

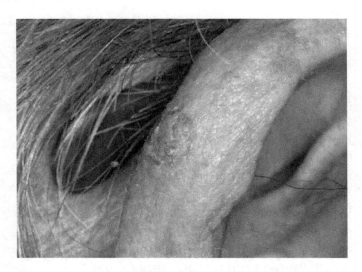

Image courtesy of The Primary Care Dermatology Society (PCDS)

An example of hyperkeratotic actinic keratosis with a raised scaly surface.

Pigmented actinic keratosis – these present as areas of hyperpigmented scaly skin which are sometimes also known as brown actinic keratosis. These can be mistaken for sun spots but can often be differentiated by the presence of rough skin on the pigmentation.

Actinic chelitis – this is an actinic keratosis which occurs on the lip, usually on the lower lip.

The Biopsy

Usually, your doctor, especially if you're seeing a dermatologist, can diagnose or rule out actinic keratosis just by examining it. However, your doctor may decide to biopsy the lesion to get a firm diagnosis and rule out early stages of either basal cell carcinoma or squamous cell carcinoma. Certain types of lesions, such as Bowenoid actinic keratosis or Lichenoid keratosis, mimic these skin cancers in their early stages. Often, it's best to err on the side of caution and send a sample of the lesion to the pathology lab.

Your doctor may choose to remove the entire lesion or just a small portion of the lesion in order to get a sample for the pathology lab. A local anesthetic will be used to numb the area and is usually very effective. Depending on the sensitivity of the area and the type of anesthetic used, you may feel nothing at all, a slight stinging or just a painless scraping or pressure.

It takes just a moment to get the biopsy sample and the area will just require a topical antibiotic and a small bandage. Once the anesthetic wears off, you may feel some burning or stinging in the area for a day or so, but the whole process is fairly painless.

If your doctor doesn't volunteer the information, you'll want to ask when he expects to get the results from the pathology lab. If there is a lab onsite, it often takes less than forty-eight hours to get results. An off-site laboratory may take as long as two weeks. It's helpful to know beforehand so that you aren't overly concerned or anxious about not getting the results right away.

Your doctor may choose to remove the entire lesion right away, before waiting for the laboratory results. This shouldn't make you more anxious. It isn't necessarily a sign that your doctor is concerned about the outcome. Usually it's simply a matter of efficiency. An actinic keratosis is going to have to be removed at any rate and might just as well be done while you're there, as opposed to doing it at the follow-up appointment once the lab work is back.

Whether your doctor chooses to biopsy the lesion or is comfortable diagnosing and removing it without a biopsy, he will likely discuss ongoing treatment options with you and give you some information on preventing more lesions. As we've said, and as your doctor will likely tell you, once you've had one actinic keratosis, chances are very high that you will continue to get them. However, the goal will be to do all that you can to keep the number of lesions as low as possible.

Fortunately, there's a great deal that you can do to improve your outcome and reduce the number of actinic keratoses that you get in the future. Some of those things will involve ongoing medical treatments and some will be preventive measures that you can take yourself. We'll discuss all of these in detail in the next section.

Chapter 3 – Removal and Treatment of Actinic Keratosis

Once a diagnosis of actinic keratosis has been made and any biopsies done (if determined necessary by your physician), the next order of business will be to remove the lesions(s) and/or begin a course of topical treatment.

The two main types of treatment for actinic keratosis consist of topical and surgical procedures and often they're used together because attacking actinic keratosis from several angles is often more effective than simply treating it with one.

The main thing that you need to do is see a medical professional in order to get diagnosed with actinic keratosis prior to beginning treatment. After you discover exactly what type of actinic keratosis you have, you can then discuss treatment options with your doctor.

Most topical treatments are finished within just a few weeks and some removal treatments, such as chemical peels, take care of the problem with just one treatment.

Different treatments have different side effects but most are extremely mild and don't cause permanent damage. Be aware that many of these treatments do cause sun sensitivity even after your treatments are over and that you should be very careful when going out in the sun.

The only other common side effect is skin irritation including redness or flaking, but that really is the goal; you want the actinic keratosis to flake and then come off so that healthy new skin can grow.

Again, you first need an accurate diagnosis and then you can take what you're about to learn and use it to discuss treatment options with your physician.

Because there are several that work well together, it's important to talk about your options with your medical professional and make an educated decision together. Getting a diagnosis of actinic keratosis is scary, but knowing your options and the efficacy of each one will help you to take control of your situation and make positive choices.

Methods for Removing Actinic Keratoses

There is no one removal technique preferred by all physicians. The type of lesion you have and the number of total lesions has much to do with the method of removal. The biopsy results and your doctor's expectations as far as prognosis are also a deciding factor.

Your doctor may well invite you to weigh in on the removal method you prefer. He should explain the pros and cons of each, but we'll explain them here so that you have some idea of what to expect and which method or methods you might prefer to use.

Cryotherapy

If there is only one lesion or a small number of lesions, many physicians choose to remove them via cryotherapy. Cryotherapy is simply using liquid nitrogen to freeze and "kill" the lesion. Liquid nitrogen freezes at a temperature of -195 degrees F and keratinocytes die when the reach a temperature of -40 to -50 degrees F, making cryosurgery a very efficient means of removal.

45

Your doctor may choose to use a cotton-tip applicator dipped in liquid nitrogen, but it's far more common to use a handheld liquid nitrogen spray applicator, especially in a very small or tight area.

The handheld spray device emits continuous bursts of the liquid nitrogen in a very tiny stream, which allows the physician to carefully control the area being treated. This is important, because if the skin in the immediate area is affected, a whitish scarring may occur and is often very visible on very light-skinned patients.

The possibility of scarring is generally quite small, however, as long as you're being treated by a doctor who is familiar with actinic keratosis and has performed cryosurgery regularly.

The cryosurgery procedure takes less than a minute and no local anesthetic or anesthesia is required.

You may feel some burning with the cryosurgery, both during the procedure and for a few hours afterward, but it's nothing to be alarmed about.

Your doctor will usually cover the lesion with a small bandage and ask that you keep it clean and dry. You may be asked not to shower for 24 hours after the procedure. Within a few days, the lesion will dry out and fall off on its own. You may see a slight red spot for a short time, but healing is usually completed within four or five days on the face and within a week to two weeks on the trunk, arms or legs.

One treatment may be enough to get rid of lesions on your face. Up to four weeks of treatment may be required for treatments on your arms, trunk or legs. Your doctor will determine how many times he wants to treat you. Cryosurgery is often used in conjunction with 5-FU (fluorouracil 0.5% cream); if so, it's typically done 1-2 weeks after beginning treatment with the fluorouracil.

There are few side effects associated with cryosurgery, but you may experience:

- Soreness
- Redness
- Itching
- Whitening of nearby healthy skin
- Minor scarring

Application of Vitamin E cream may be helpful to speed healing, reduce itching and reduce the chance of scarring. Avoid very hot baths and showers for the first couple of days, as the tender skin can burn easily. However, a warm bath may be soothing.

There are a couple of reasons why your doctor may suggest using an alternative method of removal. Cryosurgery is only recommended for a single lesion or just a few small lesions.

It's also not always the best method for those patients who have or have had diabetes, poor circulation, Hepatitis-C, some lymphoid disorders or any kind of connective tissue disease, as those patients carry a cryoprotein that impairs healing.

Your doctor may also choose another method of removal if your lesion is on your lower leg, as wounds below the knee tend to heal slowly and an ulcer may develop after using cryosurgery.

However, cryosurgery is the fastest and one of the most effective methods of removing actinic keratoses and will probably be the recommended means of removal for most patients.

According to one study, the cure rate for actinic keratoses treated with cryosurgery is between 75-99% (Lubritz RR, Smolewski SA 1982). The length of the actual treatment has a good deal to do with the cure rate according to one group of researchers, who found that lesions treated for five seconds only had a 39% cure rate, while those treated for 20 seconds or more had a cure rate of 89%. (Thai KE, Fergin P, Freeman M, Vinciullo C, Francis D, Spelman L, et al. 2004)

If your doctor proposes using cryosurgery to remove your lesion(s), be sure to ask how long the liquid nitrogen will be applied to the lesion(s).

Curettage or Traditional Surgery

Many physicians still prefer curettage, or cutting away the lesion, as a means of removing an actinic keratosis. This is most often the case when the doctor has decided to do a biopsy of the lesion, since he will already be scraping or snipping a small portion for testing. However, many physicians prefer this method even when a biopsy is not required.

The procedure is done in the doctor's office as an outpatient and usually involves using a local anesthetic to numb the area.

The doctor uses a small curette or scalpel-like tool to scrape away the lesion, leaving the normal skin intact.

The procedure only takes a few minutes and is relatively painless. You may feel a slight stinging or burning sensation or nothing at all. The area will then be covered with a small bandage for the first 24-48 hours.

There are no side effects to curettage, but there are some downsides. There is some chance of scarring, and some normal tissue may be damaged during the procedure. Curettage may also require additional treatment with a topical medicine and recurrence is more likely than with other methods of removal.

If you're taking blood thinners, have diabetes or are a hemophiliac, curettage may not be offered as an option for you because of the possibility of excessive bleeding and slow healing.

Chemical Peel

Using the method of chemical peeling to remove actinic keratoses is less common than is cryosurgery, but there are several instances where it may be a better option.

Chemical peeling is preferred by some physicians for treating actinic keratoses located on the face. In particular, actinic cheilitis (actinic keratosis on the lower lip) is often best-treated with chemical peeling.

A chemical peel involves applying trichloroacetic acid (TCA), or a combination of chemicals including TCA. This is usually Jessner's solution, which contains resorcinol, lactic acid, and salicylic acid in ethanol. (Lawrence N, Cox SE, Cockerell CJ, Freeman RG, Cruz PD Jr 1995)

The solution is applied directly to the lesion. The physician uses a special dropper-like applicator or a tool similar to a very small paintbrush to apply the chemicals only to the affected area.

The procedure only takes a few minutes and your doctor will apply a local anesthetic; either a topical cream or a numbing shot. You may feel just a tinge of heat or stinging, but the procedure should be relatively painless.

You will have some redness after the procedure, but this usually only lasts from a few hours to a couple of days. Over the course of about a week, the top layers of skin will slough off and be replaced with new skin, so there may be a pink tinge to the skin for a short time as the area heals.

Here are some of the common side effects from chemical peels:

- Pain and burning
- Redness
- Irritation
- Mild swelling
- Temporary discoloration

Many patients report that applying Vitamin E cream to the area treated with a chemical peel helped to speed healing and reduce tenderness but you should speak with your doctor about this before you try it yourself (Cole MD 2013). Your doctor may prefer to have you use a prescription cream to speed healing and prevent infection.

Chemical peeling is usually advised when the actinic keratosis is level with the skin rather than a raised spot, when close to the eye and when a lesion or lesions cover an area too large for the use of cryosurgery.

Results with chemical peeling are generally excellent and are comparable to the use of fluorouracil 0.5% cream, which is considered the standard of topical treatments for actinic keratosis. The advantage of chemical peeling over fluorouracil 0.5% cream is that there is usually only one treatment needed. (Lawrence

N, Cox SE, Cockerell CJ, Freeman RG, Cruz PD Jr 1995)

We'll discuss fluorouracil 0.5% cream in greater detail in the next section.

Laser Surgery

Laser surgery or laser treatment of the affected area is less commonly used in treating actinic keratosis, but it does have its place.

Laser therapy consists of using an erbium YAG or carbon dioxide laser to cut through your tissue in order to remove the lesion without causing bleeding or more than minor pain (Actinic Keratosis 2013). You may receive local anesthesia but it's not typically painful. As with a chemical peel, you'll be receiving this treatment in a doctor or medical professional's office or hospital.

There are few side effects to laser surgery. The area may be red and tender for a couple of days, but there is typically very little scarring. Your doctor may suggest a healing cream be applied for a week or two.

Typically you'll only receive one laser surgery to remove your actinic keratoses. Since it's great for use in small or narrow spaces, laser surgery is a good alternative for use on the face, scalp, or other areas that are difficult to reach with other treatments.

Laser surgery is often used in conjunction with other treatments including 5-FU, simply because, as we've already discussed, with actinic keratosis, more is frequently better. 5-FU or Fluorouracil 5% is a topical chemotherapy treatment.

Photodynamic Therapy

Also known as PDT, phototherapy, photo-chemotherapy, blue light treatment or photo-radiation therapy, photodynamic therapy consists of applying a chemical, often Levulan or Kerastick, to your lesions, then allowing it to incubate for anywhere from a few minutes to a few hours (Habif, TP 2009).The area is then exposed to an extremely powerful light that activates the acid and destroys the actinic keratosis when the acid interacts with oxygen.

One of the advantages of photodynamic therapy is that the destruction is selective; it does very little harm to the surrounding healthy tissue. It also has no known long-term side effects, is less invasive than cryotherapy or curettage, causes little or no scarring and is usually one of the least expensive methods of removal.

Photodynamic therapy is most effective on thin layers of skin so if your lesions are thick, you may receive more than one treatment, or you may need to combine photodynamic therapy with other forms of treatment. Either way, it's often an extremely effective procedure for treatment of actinic keratosis.

There are a few reasons why photodynamic therapy may not be an option for you. First, it's important to remember that light therapy is part of the treatment process. If light can't reach the area, photodynamic therapy won't be among your treatment choices.

If you're one of those rare people who are allergic to porphyrins, a class of pigments that includes chlorophyll and heme, you can't receive photodynamic therapy safely.

Photosensitivity is also possible and sunscreen won't protect you so you'll need to cover up when you go outside and avoid the sun as much as feasible. Indirect light is important though because it helps your system break actinic keratosis down.

After a photodynamic therapy treatment, it's important that you don't use any high-heat devices such as the helmet-style hairdryers in beauty salons. That type of heat can actually reactivate the chemicals in your bloodstream and cause burning or redness. Use low heat instead for up to 30 days after receiving treatment.

Topical Treatments for Actinic Keratosis

As we've discussed, there are several topical treatments for actinic keratosis and they're most commonly used in conjunction with one of the removal methods. However, some doctors choose to restrict treatment to topical methods and do so with good results. The number of lesions you have and their severity will determine whether that's a good treatment option for you.

Fluorouracil 5%

Also known by the names 5-FU, Carac, Fluoroplex, Efudex and 5-Fluorouracil, this topical cream is actually a form of chemotherapy and is the most common treatment for actinic keratosis. It's an anti-metabolite, which means that it stops the growth of cancer cells by altering the process by which cells make DNA and RNA (ribonucleic acid; acts as a messenger carrying instructions from your DNA). The abnormal cells can no longer grow on the top layer of your skin.

Frequency and Efficacy

5-FU is typically applied in an ointment or liquid suspension at 0.5-5% concentration twice daily for 2-4 weeks. Lesions generally heal within two weeks after concluding treatment and there is rarely any scarring.

If you have any of the following conditions, you need to make sure that your doctor is aware of them before starting this medication:

- Allergies
- Medical conditions such as kidney or liver disease, diabetes, congestive heart failure, gout or infections of any sort
- If you've been treated with any other type of chemotherapy
- If you've ever been diagnosed with dihydropyrimidine dehydrogenase deficiency (DPD). This is the enzyme that your body uses to metabolize, or get rid of this chemical and if you don't have it, you can become toxic on 5-FU and develop serious side effects.

- If you're pregnant, nursing, or considering becoming pregnant in the future
- If you're taking any medications

There are a few drugs that 5-FU may interact with, so it's crucial that your doctor knows about these:

- Coumadin (aka warfarin)
- Vitamin E
- NSAIDs including acetaminophen, ibuprofen, or naproxen
- Ticlid (ticlopidine)
- Plavix (clopidogrel)
- Cold, flu, migraine, fever or allergy medications
- Seizure medications

Fluorouracil Side Effects
- Swelling and/or redness
- Burning
- Sensitivity to touch
- Itching
- Sensitivity to sun
- Skin discoloration

Because of the high success rate with fluorouracil, many doctors consider it the best choice among topical treatments and it's likely that this medication will be offered as a treatment option.

Discuss any concerns you may have and be sure to ask plenty of questions before consenting to treatment.

Imiquimod

Also known as Aldara, Zyclara, and Beseina, this is another topical treatment that is proven effective against actinic keratosis. Imiquimod is one of the top go-to treatments for people who can't have surgery. It comes in a cream that contains either 5% or 3.75% imiquimod and works by stimulating the immune response. Specifically, it promotes the production of interferon, the chemical that your body uses to destroy cancerous and precancerous cells.

Frequency and Efficacy

Imiquimod is generally used twice weekly for four to sixteen weeks and works well for about 80% of patients who use it, though only about 7% of people who use it on their hands or arms experience total clearing (Love WE, et al. 2009). It's best used in conjunction with other treatments because you can't apply it more frequently than twice per week without significantly increasing the risk of toxicity and side effects.

Side Effects and Warnings
As with 5-FU, tell your doctor if:

- You're taking any medications
- Have any medical conditions
- Are pregnant, nursing, or considering becoming pregnant

Though most people tolerate imiquimod very well, you may still experience a few side effects such as:

- Redness
- Scabbing
- Crusting
- Sun sensitivity
- Skin discoloration
- In relatively rare conditions, ulcerations

Diclofenac
Though diclofenac, aka Solaraze gel, is used with less success and therefore less frequently, it's a good treatment to use in conjunction with

other treatments. It's a non-steroidal anti-inflammatory (NSAID) that is works in conjunction with hyaluronic acid, a naturally-occurring transport agent and moisturizer found within your body.

Diclofenac works to prevent inflammation so most people don't have any side effects. The hyaluronic acid delays uptake so higher dosages can be tolerated. This cream is used frequently for people who simply can't tolerate any other forms of treatment for their actinic keratosis.

Frequency and Efficacy
Diclofenac is typically used at a 3% dosage in a 2.5% hyaluronic gel and is used daily for up to 60 days. It has limited success when used independently and there are few studies on this medication as yet.

Ingenol Mebutate

This topical gel, used under the brand name Picato, was only approved for treatment of actinic keratosis in 2012 and is still not widely used, possibly because there are only limited studies on its effectiveness and long term effects.

61

The few studies on ingenol mebutate that do exist are promising, so it's possible that we'll see an increase in the popularity of ingenol mebutate. IF your doctor is one who favors trying newer treatment protocols, he may suggest using ingenol mebutate if other methods have been less successful than desired.

Frequency and Efficacy

Ingenol mebutate is used in either .015% or .05% concentrations and effectively treats actinic keratosis in just two to three days.

The dosage that you are prescribed will be dependent upon the location of your actinic keratosis. The .015% concentration is typically used on your face or scalp one time per day for three days. The .05% concentration is usually used on the trunk and extremities once daily for just two days.

Side Effects

There are only a few side effects associated with ingenol mebutate and they include:

- Skin irritation or redness
- Scaling
- Crusting
- Flaking
- Swelling

- Itching

Side effects are fairly rare and usually minor because this treatment is generally well-tolerated; in fact, it's often used for people who can't tolerate other treatments.

Regardless of which treatment options you and your doctor decide to use, it's important that the decision be a joint one. This is your body, your health and your future, so don't be shy or self-conscious about giving your input. Your doctor would do the same if he were in your situation.

When discussing the options for treatment, be sure to express your concerns, share your research, ask plenty of questions and be open about any preferences you may have for one treatment option over another.

Your doctor may have specific and very valid reasons for preferring a treatment that causes you concern, but may not explain those reasons unless you talk openly about what's concerning you. An explanation of his reasoning may put your mind at ease, or, once hearing your thoughts, he may be perfectly happy to use another course of treatment that is considered just as effective.

The important thing is to decide on a means of treatment together and get all of your questions answered so that you can proceed confidently and with as little anxiety as possible.

Follow-Up Treatment for Actinic Keratosis

Once your initial lesions have been treated, either by removal, topical medication or some combination of the two, your follow-up treatment will consist primarily of regular skin examinations.

Remember that the more lesions you have, the more likely it is that one or more of them will develop into squamous cell carcinoma, so you will need to have your skin examined on a regular basis to keep those numbers low.

Initially, your doctor may ask you to schedule an exam every few months or even more frequently. Depending on how often new lesions are found and on their severity, you may be able to stretch out those examinations to every six months or even annual visits.

64

However, you are more likely to find lesions as you age, especially once you reach sixty years of age, so it may be necessary to have your skin examined several times a year.

While regular skin exams and any necessary repeated treatments are the basis of your medical treatment, there are many very effective and very important things that you can do yourself to prevent additional actinic keratoses and to lessen the chances that you may face cancerous lesions later on.

These steps will not only help ensure the best outcome and continued good health, they'll also help you to feel empowered rather than helpless. That's essential to someone who's received a diagnosis of actinic keratosis.

Chapters Five and Six are devoted to explaining those steps and getting you started on a proactive treatment plan of your own.

Chapter 4 Squamous Cell Carcinoma

So far, we've discussed the fact that actinic keratosis is, for the most part, an aesthetic condition that is typically harmless. That remains true but we felt that in order to provide you with as much information as possible, it was only responsible to include a section in this book about squamous cell carcinoma, the type of cancer most often related to actinic keratosis.

Though actinic keratosis only progresses to cancer about ten-percent of the time, it's crucial for you to know the signs and symptoms in order to catch and treat it early.

What is Squamous Cell Carcinoma?

Squamous cell carcinoma is the second most common type of skin cancer. It forms in the flat squamous cells that make up most of the outer layers of your skin (Actinic Keratosis 2013). It is highly treatable with early detection.

According to the Skin Cancer Foundation, about 700,000 new cases of squamous cell carcinoma are diagnosed in the US each year, resulting in about 2,500 deaths. Of those, about 40-60 percent of squamous cell carcinoma occurrences begin as actinic keratosis. (Skin Cancer Foundation n.d.)

Since about 58 million people in the US are currently dealing with actinic keratosis and squamous cell carcinoma is so easily treatable, it's important to to know all that you can about this form of skin cancer. (Squamous Cell Carcinoma n.d.)

What is Bowen's Disease?
Bowen's disease or Bowenoid actinic keratosis, used to be categorized similarly to actinic keratosis – a separate condition that was simply a risk factor that could lead to the development of squamous cell carcinoma. Now it's recognized as the early, non-invasive stage of squamous cell carcinoma. It manifests as reddish brown scaly patch on your skin that you may mistake for psoriasis or dry skin.

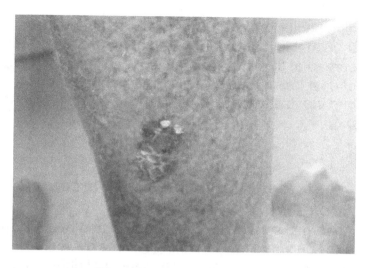

Image courtesy of The Primary Care Dermatology Society (PCDS)

Bowen's disease or Bowenoid actinic keratosis on the calf. Note the red color and scaly patches.

Though it's usually caused by sun damage and appears on areas of skin most often exposed to the sun, Bowen's disease can appear anywhere on your body. Genetics, toxins, radiation, exposure to arsenic, and even the human Papillomavirus can cause it.

Left untreated, Bowen's disease may invade deeper skin or tissue structures and may spread. Follow the same recommendations for avoiding Bowen's disease as you do for avoiding squamous cell carcinoma. There is also a vaccine for HPV available to females age 9-26 that is highly effective in preventing the spread of the virus, which also reduces your risk of developing Bowen's disease, genital warts and cervical cancer. (Skin Cancer Foundation n.d.)

What Does Squamous Cell Carcinoma Look Like?

Abnormal squamous cells develop and begin to grow uncontrollably, forming lesions on your skin's surface that manifest in several different ways. When they develop from actinic keratosis, obviously, they're going to look just like the rest of your actinic keratosis spots in the beginning. You should see your physician if the spots change in any of the following ways:

- Shape

- Size

- Color

- Texture

- Any other change in appearance

- Bleeding

- Itching

70

- Swelling
- Pain

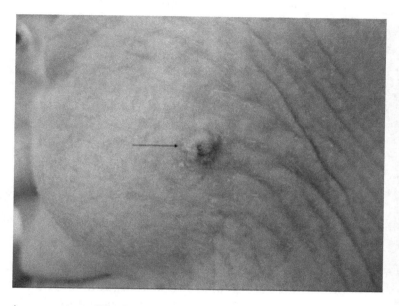

Image courtesy of The Primary Care Dermatology Society (PCDS)

An image of squamous cell carcinoma. Note multiple colors and a rough, raised surface.

Squamous cell carcinoma can develop anywhere on your body, including inside your nose or mouth, but is most common on areas that are regularly exposed to the sun. Just as with actinic keratosis, squamous cell carcinoma generally occurs on your face, ears, lips, neck, hands, arms, legs and bald head. A good clue that an area may be at risk is that there is already sun damage in the form of spots, wrinkles or actinic keratosis.

Actinic keratosis is often referred to as a precancerous condition because of the chance that it may develop into squamous cell carcinoma or another type of cancer, but that doesn't mean that it's going to. As we've already discussed, the odds are only about 10 percent that it will. If it does progress, though, it can become disfiguring.

Though squamous cell carcinoma grows faster than basal cell carcinoma, the other most common type of skin cancer, it can still move fairly slowly, so the chances of curing it before it moves to other parts of your body are very good, as long as it's detected early on.

Actinic keratosis, as we've already discussed, is simply a rough spot on your skin that stays relatively flat and consistent in appearance and doesn't change. Squamous cell carcinoma may start out in the same way but it changes in appearance and may manifest as any of the following:

- Red, raised, scaly patch of skin with irregular borders. May bleed.

- An open sore that refuses to heal.

- A wart-like growth that may get crusty or bleed.

- A horn-like growth above the skin.

- An elevated ring of skin with a depressed center that sometimes bleeds. This type may grow rapidly.

- Any change in an existing actinic keratosis, wart, mole, freckle or other skin anomaly.

What Causes Squamous Cell Carcinoma?

When your squamous cells are normal, the new cells push the old ones to the top so that they can just slough off and be replaced. When there is a disruption in the DNA strand, the cells begin to pile up on top of each other and grow uncontrollably without sloughing off like they're supposed to. The disruption in the DNA sequence causes the cells to reproduce more irregular cells and the cancer spreads. (Skin Cancer Foundation n.d.)

The most common cause of this disruption or damage to your squamous cells is caused by the UV rays found in sunshine or in tanning bed bulbs. Remember though that squamous cell carcinoma can develop anywhere, even on your genitals or anus; areas that aren't typically exposed to sunlight. That means that other factors such as injury, exposure to environmental toxins or perhaps a weak immune system may also cause damage your squamous cells.

Risk Factors for Squamous Cell Carcinoma

Though anybody can develop skin cancer, having at least one actinic keratosis does increase your risk and the risk rises with the number of lesions. That said, the risk factors for squamous cell carcinoma are much the same as those for actinic keratosis, including:

- Being fair-skinned

- Having blue or green eyes

- Having blond or red hair

- Getting older – squamous cell carcinoma is rare before age 50 and most common in people in their 70's

- Frequent severe sunburns at a young age

- Exposure to toxic chemicals

- Long-term regular sun exposure

- Undergoing many x-rays throughout life

- Having actinic keratosis, leukoplakia or actinic cheilitis – the more lesions you have, the higher your odds that one will develop into skin cancer

- Being male – men are twice as likely to develop squamous cell carcinoma, possibly because they tend to be outside more due to employment choices

- Having already had some form of skin cancer

- People with genetic conditions that make them sensitive to UV rays

- Frequently using a tanning bed increases your odds by 2.5 percent

- Areas that have been injured by burns, cuts, ulcers, inflammation, or long-lasting sores

- People with compromised immune systems

- Genetic predisposition to skin cancer

How is Squamous Cell Carcinoma Diagnosed?

If you do find a spot that concerns you, don't wait to make an appointment with your doctor. It's better to be overly cautious than to write it off as just another, extra-scaly actinic keratosis.

If the doctor finds something that concerns him, he may take a clipping or scraping of the skin and send it off for a biopsy. This is no more involved than a biopsy for actinic keratosis, but your doctor may wait to remove the lesion completely until he has a firm diagnosis.

Treatment Options for Squamous Cell Carcinoma

When detected early and treated quickly, squamous cell carcinoma is nearly always curable. You probably won't even have much of a scar to show for your experience! If you don't catch it in time, though, it can spread to your other tissues. At that point, you're risking everything from disfigurement to death. Though squamous cell carcinoma is rarely fatal, it can happen.

Once you're diagnosed, you'll have a number of treatment options based upon how far your cancer has progressed, where it's located, how big it is and what type it is.

Nearly every option can be performed on an outpatient basis so that you go home right after the procedure takes place. Minimal pain will be involved either during or after the procedure and a local anesthetic is probably all that your doctor will use while he's removing the cancer.

Many of the same treatments that are used for actinic keratosis are also used to treat squamous cell carcinoma, including:

- Photodynamic or blue light therapy

77

- Laser surgery

- Topical medications such as 5-FU and imiquimod

- Cryosurgery

Other treatments that are commonly used include:

- Mohs surgery – one layer of skin is removed at a time and examined under the microscope until no signs of cancer are apparent in the layer removed. Typically used on cancers on the face and ears. (US National Library of Medicine and National Institutes of Health n.d.)

- Radiation – x-ray beams are aimed directly at the lesion several times per week for anywhere from one to four weeks. Treatment may even be done daily. Cure rates range from 85-95 percent. Since we know that radiation and x-rays actually cause skin cancer, this treatment is usually reserved for patients who can't undergo any of the other treatments.

- Excisional surgery – this one is exactly what the name implies. Your doctor will simply cut the entire growth, along with a bit of healthy tissue, out of the site. The wound is then stitched up and the tissue that he cut out will be sent to the lab to ensure that all cancerous cells were removed. Cure rate for excisional surgery is about 92 percent for first-time occurrences but drops to 77 percent for recurring carcinomas.

- Electro-surgery, also known as curettage or electrodessication – Your doctor will scrape off a deep layer of tissue in order to remove the growth. He'll cauterize the wound both to stop the bleeding and to kill any cancer cells left behind. This is often used on superficially invasive squamous cell carcinomas and has a cure rate of about 92 percent for this type. It's not as effective for more aggressive or invasive types of squamous cell carcinoma.

Some Final Words

Though it's unlikely that your actinic keratosis will develop into squamous cell carcinoma or any other cancer, you should still be aware that it's possible. Conduct regular self-examinations of your skin, report anything odd to your doctor and don't delay treatment if you're diagnosed with skin cancer.

Squamous cell carcinoma is one of the easiest cancers to avoid and to treat. Cure rates are extremely high and mortality rates are extremely low.

Chapter 5 Living with Actinic Keratosis

As is true with many ongoing health concerns, what you do after the diagnosis is just as important as what the doctors may do.

There are so many steps that you can take to lessen recurrence of actinic keratosis and also to lower your risk of developing cancerous lesions. You are also in charge of how you feel about life and your health from this point forward.

While everyone has the right to have some down moments, a positive attitude and optimistic outlook are critical to both your happiness and your health.

In this section, we'll look at the lifestyle changes you can make to greatly reduce your risk of actinic keratosis and skin cancer. We'll also discuss taking good care of your emotional health, which is every bit as important.

Your New Relationship with the Sun

There are several steps you can take for your health and you can take them right away. Primarily, those steps have to do with protecting yourself from sun damage, boosting your immunity and making some nutritional changes that can reduce your chances of getting more actinic keratoses.

Protecting Yourself from the Sun

The single most important thing that you can do for yourself is to protect your skin from any further sun damage. As we discussed in Chapter 1, actinic keratoses are directly caused by sun damage. The more you limit sun damage, the more you limit actinic keratosis.

Forget about Sunbathing

If you're one of the many people who don't feel attractive without a tan, you'll need to either change your feelings about pale skin or change your method of getting some color. The worst thing you can do is continue to intentionally expose yourself to the sun.

Tanning beds are not an alternative option. You get just as much harmful UV exposure through tanning beds as you do from the sun, sometimes much more.

Although self-tanning lotions and sprays used to be difficult to use and produce less than attractive results, they've come a long way in the last few years. There are several excellent products on the market that are inexpensive, easy to apply and that produce a very natural tan appearance. They also tend to smell better than the products that were available even a few years ago and most of them no longer give you that telltale odor.

If you think that self-tanning lotions take too much time, investigate the newer products. Many of them come in continuous spray form and dry very quickly. There are also daily lotions that are applied just like regular moisturizers and produce a gradual tan that is maintained in just a few minutes a day.

Self-tanning lotions may have been a joke ten years ago, but they are now used by celebrities, models and make-up artists all over the world.

If you balk at the idea of having to apply self-tanning lotion, you may want to try a spray-tanning booth. They're widely available, often in gyms and hair salons as well as fully-fledged tanning salons.

The advantages of spray tanning are that it only takes a few minutes, is very inexpensive and usually lasts a week to two weeks. The results are surprisingly natural with most spray tans and there is little to no odor. If you don't think you want to tackle self-tanning at home, this may be a great option for you.

No matter which self-tanning option you choose, you'll be making a change that can have a dramatic impact on your chances of getting more actinic keratoses.

Protect Yourself When You Must Be in the Sun

Even if you're not a sun-worshipper, you'll still spend some time in the sun and of course you should. Fresh air and being outdoors in great weather adds a lot of enjoyment to your life, especially if you have hobbies and activities that take you outside.

You don't need to give up the outdoor activities that you love and there will be times when you must be outside during the day, especially if your job requires it. But you do need to make sure that you're protected and that you use common sense.

The most important sun protection in your arsenal will be a good sunblock. You should start making it a habit to apply sunblock every morning, just as you wash your face and brush your teeth.

The higher the SPF you wear, the better. There are sunblocks that go as high as 70SPF, although research results conflict on the efficacy of anything above 50SPF. Choose a block with an SPF of 50 or more and a waterproof lotion can be a good idea to prevent perspiration, rain or a little splashing from washing your protection away.

Generally, waterproof and higher SPF lotions tend to be quite thick and can be difficult to rub in without a telltale whitish film on the skin. If this is something that will give you an excuse to skip your sunblock, then by all means use the highest SPF oil or clear gel that you can find, but be sure to reapply frequently as per the package directions. It's better to wear a lower SPF or to have to reapply it frequently than to wear no protection at all.

When applying the sunblock, be generous and be sure to apply it to areas that are sometimes forgotten, such as your ears, the part in your hair (or your scalp if you are bald or balding), your nose, eyebrows, the back of your neck and so on.

Some lotions require you to reapply the sunblock every hour or two (according to directions) if you're out in the sun for an extended time, if you swim or get wet or if you're doing strenuous work or exercise. For that reason, it's a good idea to keep an extra bottle in your purse, your car or somewhere else convenient. There has been a rise in the popularity of once-a-day sun tan lotions which can keep you protected for around 6 hours so it's worth investigating these too.

Don't forget to apply sunblock to your lips as well, or at least a lip balm that contains sunscreen. This is especially true if you had an actinic cheilitis (an actinic keratosis on the lower lip) but it applies to everyone, male or female. Men, there are plenty of lip balms that are unnoticeable, so please don't skip this step.

Keep in mind that you're exposed to harmful UV rays even on cloudy and overcast days. This is why it's essential to make sunblock a daily habit that comes naturally, regardless of the weather.

It's also important to remember that you are exposed to UV rays through window glass, including the windshield of your car and your car's windows. Essentially, if you can feel the sun's heat on your skin, you are exposing it to damaging UV rays, so pay heed.

Avoid the Strongest Rays of the Day

UV rays are at their most plentiful between the hours of 10am and 4pm, no matter where you live. However, the closer you are to the equator, the stronger the sun's rays are, even before 10am and after 4pm.

If at all possible, avoid being outside for too long during these hours. If it's not possible to avoid the sun during this period, it's a good idea to wear additional sun protection along with your sunblock.

Wear Additional Protection

Hats that shade your face, long sleeves and sunglasses all provide an extra measure of protection, though they're not very effective alone. Darker clothes provide more protection than do white or light-colored clothing and thicker hats made of cloth are better than straw or other open weaves. Keep in mind, though, that clothing and hats only add about 30-60 minutes of extra protection and they are not a substitute for sunblock.

A Word about Vitamin D

Our bodies don't manufacture Vitamin D independently; they produce it by converting it from the sun's rays.

Vitamin D is essential to good health, but if you're wearing sunblock every day and limiting your time in the sun, you're likely to develop a Vitamin D deficiency.

When you lack enough Vitamin D, you can become fatigued, experience bone and joint pain and even become depressed. The long term effects include osteoporosis or bone weakness, tooth loss and chronic pain. (MF 2010)

While you can get some Vitamin D from foods such as milk, cheese, yogurt and some fish, it can be difficult to get an adequate supply from diet alone if you don't care for dairy foods or live in an area where winters are long or the weather is gray and overcast much of the time. It's a good idea to take a Vitamin D supplement daily to ensure that your body has what it needs. How much you need will depend on your diet, how much time you do spend outdoors, your climate and your weight. Ask your doctor for dosage recommendations.

Of all the things that you can and should do for your health after a diagnosis of actinic keratosis, protecting yourself from the sun is the most vital.

While it can be hard to adjust your habits and lifestyle, especially if you've always been an outdoorsy person, there is no treatment that can prevent a recurrence of actinic keratosis. Only prevention can do that for you, so please don't neglect these steps to safeguard your health.

Chapter 6 Boosting Your Immune System Naturally

Aside from protecting yourself from further damage from the sun's rays, boosting your immune system is one of the most important things you can do to help prevent additional actinic keratoses and the possible squamous cell carcinoma that can result.

Why You Need to Boost Your Immune System

Many people mistakenly think of their immune systems simply as a shield against colds, viruses and diseases. The truth is that your immune system is at work every day, battling internal parasites, environmental and food toxins, free radicals, inflammation, stress and a host of other problems.

Your immune system is your body's first defense against both actinic keratosis and any form of cancer, but our lifestyles, diets and environments all work against optimal immune function.

It's essential, then, to do everything that you can to enable your immune system to function the way it was designed. Fortunately, that's not very difficult.

Despite the ads and commercials hoping to sell you a magic, immunity-boosting supplement, truly effective action has to take a 360-degree approach.

No system in your body is wholly independent and your immune system involves several other systems, including your endocrine and digestive systems. By taking steps to improve the function of both your immune systems and its support network, you can greatly improve your overall health and reduce your risk of developing not only actinic keratoses but several forms of cancer.

There are several steps you can take to return your immune system to maximal function. They include:

- Quitting smoking

- Reducing stress

- Getting adequate sleep

- Getting regular moderate exercise

- Improving digestive health

- Cleansing the liver

- Eating an immune-friendly diet

We're going to discuss each of these in depth. You'll find that the steps involved are not difficult and are actually quite often pleasurable.

You don't need to adopt every single habit or implement every change at once. Some may not apply to you or may be things you're already doing. Regardless, even if you do decide you want to do every single one of these suggestions, you don't need to make yourself frantic trying to do everything at once. In fact, that would likely cause you a good amount of stress and reducing stress is one of your objectives!

Instead, choose one thing to do at a time, or even one thing from each category. Then add another each week or every other week until each is a habit.

One of the important side benefits of taking your immune health into your own hands is that it takes away the sense of powerlessness that often accompanies a diagnosis of actinic keratosis. Taking very proactive steps to improve your prognosis puts you in a position of being in charge of your own health to a great extent and the psychological benefit is as great as the medical.

Step One: Boosting Your Immune System by Quitting Smoking

If you smoke cigarettes, you already know the dangers of this terribly addictive product. No doubt, you've heard all of the lectures and read all of the alarming reports that you care to about your high risk of developing several cancers, including lung cancer, cancer of the mouth and throat cancer.

Smoking also has a direct impact on your immune system. There are 7,000 chemicals in every cigarette, 65 of them known to be carcinogenic. Your immune system is hard at work battling every single toxin, every single day. This puts a severe drain on your immune system's resources and causes widespread, chronic inflammation. In short, your body is so busy fighting off the cigarettes that it doesn't have the wherewithal for preventing actinic keratoses or squamous cell carcinoma.

Chemicals in tobacco smoke cause inflammation and cell damage, and can weaken the immune system. The body makes white blood cells to respond to injuries, infections, and cancers. White blood cell counts stay high while smoking continues, meaning the body is constantly fighting against the damage caused by smoking which can lead to disease in almost any part of the body. (A Report of the Surgeon General: How Tobacco Smoke Causes Disease -The Biology and Behavioral Basis for Smoking-Attributable Disease 2014)

Quitting smoking is an incredibly difficult task. Smoking is one of the most powerful chemical and psychological addictions in existence and has been compared to heroin in the strength of its hold on users.

However, people quit smoking every day and you can do it, as well. If you've tried unsuccessfully to quit before, take heart in knowing that very few people who have quit were able to do so the first time.

There are a number of methods that have been shown to be successful in quitting smoking. There are many products available to help you quit. These include nicotine replacement patches and gums, prescription medications such as Chantix and some anti-depressants and electronic cigarettes (though the jury is out on whether electronic cigarettes may also cause problems). What works for one person may not work for you and you may even need to use more than one to finally quit smoking.

Some people are more successful with old, tried-and-true methods such as quitting cold turkey or tapering down on their own, joining a support group and even hypnosis.

Regardless of the method or methods you choose, choose to quit. Even if you take every other step in this book to boost your immunity, if you are continuing to smoke it will place such a burden on your immune system that it will not be able to operate on anything close to a highly functional level.

Chronic inhalation of cigarette smoke alters a wide range of immunological functions, including innate and adaptive immune responses. It has been speculated that many of the health consequences of chronic inhalation of cigarette smoke might be due to its adverse effects on the immune system. (Sopori 2002)

Additionally, a diagnosis of actinic keratosis may not be a clear indicator that you will get skin cancer, but it is a clear indicator that you are predisposed to that possibility. Why would you do everything you can to prevent one cancer while you continue to put yourself at very high risk of developing another?

In the vein of searching for the silver lining, you can use your actinic keratosis as an impetus to finally commit to quitting smoking once and for all. It's one of the best examples we can imagine of turning something potentially bad into something very, very good.

Step Two: Boosting Your Immune System by Reducing Stress

Everyone knows that stress is bad for us and the more we learn about our bodies, the more we understand just exactly how harmful stress really is.

You most likely know that it can cause headaches, moodiness and even heart attacks, but research is showing now that stress is also linked to cancer, diabetes and even skin conditions such as actinic keratosis.

When you become stressed, your immune system is suppressed and simply can't function properly. It can't fight diseases and it can't build new cells to replace the ones that are lost every day just through aging. Let's look at some of the effects that stress has on the immune system, how that affects your health and what you can do to decrease stress in order to stay healthy.

Stress and Your Immune System

In order to understand how stress directly
suppresses your immune system, you need to
have a general understanding of how your body
fights disease. Your immune system's front line
soldiers are white blood cells that circulate
throughout your body, looking for pathogens
and cells compromised by disease or injury.
There are essentially two types of cells and
each fights sickness in distinctly different ways.

B-Cells make and release antibodies that
circulate in the fluid around **all** cells in order to
destroy pathogens before they can infect the
healthy cells.

T-Cells jump in when a cell becomes damaged
or endangered; by latching onto the cell,
multiplying, and then killing the cell. (Kour K,
Pandey A, Suri KA, Satti NK, Gupta KK, Bani S.
2009)

When our bodies are stressed, we release
several hormones, including adrenaline and
cortisol, as a sort of alarm system to get the
body ready to deal with danger and avoid or
heal injury. The fight or flight response is
triggered and your body is doing what it can to

ensure survival. (E.Miller, Susan C Segerstrom and Gregory. n.d.)

Adrenaline increases blood pressure, increases your heart rate and gives you a burst of energy. It also increases cholesterol, which we know can lead to cardiovascular disease and atherosclerosis or hardening of the arteries.

Cortisol increases glucose levels and enhances your brain's ability to use glucose in order to function just a little bit better. It also suppresses non-essential functions such as the release of B-cells and T-cells, thus decreasing the body's ability to fight disease and sickness.

This may not have much of an impact short-term but if your immune system is suppressed by these natural corticosteroids for an extended period of time, it's fairly obvious what the negative implications to your health would be.

In addition to having this direct impact on your immune system, there are other indirect ways that stress decreases your body's ability to keep you healthy.

For instance, stress suppresses the digestive process, which is responsible for nutrient absorption. Your body uses antioxidants and other vitamins and minerals to fight free radicals, nourish your cells and keep your body healthy in general.

We'll talk more in-depth about immunity and the digestive system later on in this chapter, but when stress suppresses your digestive system, you aren't able to absorb all of the nutrients you're eating, especially vitamins and antioxidants. This can impair your immune system even further and creates a cycle that's difficult to break if changes aren't made.

Stress hormones affect mood, sleep, memory, weight loss or gain and just about everything else going on in your body. This cycle of destruction goes on and on simply because each function of your body is linked to so many other functions. In short, chronic stress destroys your health.

Obviously, it's impossible to eliminate stress from your life entirely, but there are many changes that you can make to your lifestyle that will help to reduce it significantly.

Ways to Reduce or Eliminate Everyday Stress

Exercise
One of the best ways to release stress from your body is to exercise. A combination of cardio and strength training will not only help keep you in peak physical condition but will also help reduce stress by releasing mood-lifting hormones such as dopamine and serotonin.

If you haven't tried it, you may want to look into one of the many forms of yoga. Classes are plentiful and inexpensive and yoga has been shown to help relieve stress by utilizing stretching, deep breathing and focus.

Meditation
Meditation is a great way to clear your head and regain focus. There are many different ways to meditate so find a way that works for you and make it a daily habit.

Meditation doesn't require a great deal of time; even ten to twenty minutes is often enough to add a period of calm and stillness to your day. It's also helpful to learn some form of meditation that you can call on in times of stress, even if it's just a few simple, deep-breathing exercises.

Prayer and Faith

Some studies have shown that people who exercise some form of faith and who regularly pray according to their faith tend to feel calmer, stronger and less alone in times of trouble. Prayer has even been shown to slow the heart rate and reduce blood pressure.

Places of faith are often a good resource for support and companionship, which can also help to reduce your everyday stress levels.

Martial Arts

Many people find that learning and practicing some form of martial arts helps them to vent their frustrations and expend the excess energy that often accompanies stress and tension.

There are many forms of martial arts and one of them is likely to suit your personality, your needs and your physical condition. You might feel more comfortable with the calm, quiet movements of Tai Chi or enjoy one of the more strenuous arts such as Kung Fu or Jiu-Jitsu.

Martial arts are also a great form of exercise, so you can achieve two goals in one if your schedule is particularly tight.

Eat a Healthy Diet

When you give your body what it needs to stay healthy and fight disease, it can better deal with stress as well. We'll talk more about boosting your immunity with diet, but for the purposes of relieving stress, there are several foods that are known to help stabilize your mood and even ward off depression.

These include foods high in omega-3 fatty acids, such as cold-water fish (such as cod, haddock and salmon) as well as foods high in niacin, such as green leafy vegetables and cooked beans.

There are also several foods that help to reduce the effects of stress by providing the amino acid tryptophan. Tryptophan is used by the body to produce serotonin, which is a neurotransmitter that prompts a feeling of calm, wellbeing and happiness. (Turner EH, Loftis JM, Blackwell AD 2006)

Egg whites are highest in tryptophan per ounce, but spirulina, cod, Parmesan cheese, soybeans, turkey and cheddar cheese also contain a good amount.

Laugh

Laughter releases endorphins, those feel-good hormones that leave you relaxed and content. Even when you're feeling a bit stressed by your diagnosis, you should try to find something to laugh about at least once a day.

Watch your favorite comedy show, spend some time with an especially witty friend, or just check out your favorite funny website online. A few minutes of laughter not only release helpful hormones, but also help remind you that actinic keratosis is just one part of your life, not the center of it.

Rest

Rest isn't the same thing as sleep. Resting means regularly taking time to do something quiet and calming, to get away from your daily grind and even to be alone.

Try to schedule some down time into every day or at least several times a week. Take a long bath, curl up to read a book, go for a walk in the park or just turn off all of your electronics for a day. Sleep refreshes us physically, but rest refreshes and replenishes us mentally and emotionally.

Talk

Although you're probably greatly relieved by a diagnosis of actinic keratosis versus skin cancer, your diagnosis has had an impact on your life. It's a warning that you will have to mindful of your exposure to the sun and to paying careful attention to any changes in your skin. It's also brought you an awareness that you are at risk of developing squamous cell carcinoma.

People react in different ways to a diagnosis of actinic keratosis, but it's common to have feelings of anger, helplessness, fear and resentment toward something that has an impact on your lifestyle and your habits and that has the potential to influence your health.

It's always good to have a close friend, spouse or relative that you can talk to about your diagnosis and about the feelings it's prompted. However, some people may have a hard time understanding those feelings, since your lesions have proven to be benign rather than malignant.

It's helpful to be able to speak with someone who is also dealing with actinic keratosis. If you don't know anyone personally, there are a number of support groups and forums online that can be a great resource for information and empathy. We'll supply you with some helpful links to such sites in the resources section at the end of this book.

The important things is to be able to express your feelings and voice your fears and concerns to people who understand what you're going through or who will at least listen without discounting your feelings as unnecessary worry.

Bottling up such feelings and concerns causes a great deal of stress, even if you're not always aware of it. So does feeling that you're alone in dealing with actinic keratosis. If you don't have a close friend or family member to be that sounding board, do look into some of the options in the resources section.

Life Balance
Lack of time to enjoy life is a common problem in today's overscheduled culture. We spend so much time doing what we *have* to do that we have little time left over for doing what we *need* to do to be happy.

This causes an enormous amount of stress and fatigue, but it's a stress that is within your power to correct. Use your diagnosis as an impetus to carefully consider your life-work balance and take steps to make sure that you're not putting more on your schedule than you should.

Even if just temporarily, see what can be cut from your schedule. Do you really need to work late several times a week or is it just habit? Can you cut back on social engagements and just attend the things that have real meaning for you? Do the kids really need to have several clubs, practices and lessons per week or would all of you be happier committing to just one favorite per season?

In other words, prune your schedule down to what you absolutely must do and what you absolutely love to do. This will leave you much more time for rest, spending quality time with family and friends and creating a healthier, less stressful lifestyle.

Stress is an extremely subjective and personal thing. We all have those things, small and large, that cause us to feel anxious and overwhelmed. Some of us are go-getters who seem to thrive under deadlines and full calendars. Others feel trapped by their own schedules.

However, all of our bodies have certain physical reactions to stress, regardless of whether that stress is perceived accurately.

Take a good look at your stress level and do what you can right now to lower it as much as possible.

Step Three: Boosting Your Immunity with Adequate Sleep

We've already discussed the effect that lack of adequate sleep has on your stress level, indirectly affecting your immune system. However, numerous studies have also proven a direct link between lack of sleep and suppressed immunity.

One recent study from the University of Helsinki showed that lack of sleep for even one week actually has an impact at the genetic level.

The study observed and compared two groups of healthy young men. One group slept only four hours per night for one week and the other slept for eight hours per night for one week. Genetic testing at the end of the week showed a marked difference in the men's immune systems. Lead researcher Vilma Aho explained the initial results.

"We compared the gene expression before and after the sleep deprivation period, and focused on the genes whose behavior was most strongly altered. The expression of many genes and gene pathways related to the functions of the immune system was increased during the sleep deprivation. There was an increase in activity of

B cells which are responsible for producing antigens that contribute to the body's defensive reactions, but also to allergic reactions and asthma. This may explain the previous observations of increased asthmatic symptoms in a state of sleep deprivation." (Vilma A, et al 2013)

It's startling that only one week of sleep deprivation could cause such a marked increase in white blood cell production and activity. It's extremely common for people to skip adequate sleep during busy weeks, due to working overtime, a new baby, anxiety or even the rush of the holiday season.

But the Helsinki researchers were prompted to follow up their study with another that examined the effects of long-term sleep deprivation. What they found was even more disturbing.

What that study found was that long-term sleep deprivation, or a regular habit of sleeping less than seven hours per night, correlated with the development of inflammation-related diseases such as cardiovascular disease and Type 2 diabetes.

> *"These results corroborate the idea that sleep does not only impact brain function, but also interacts with our immune*

system and metabolism. Sleep loss causes changes to the system that regulates our immune defense. Some of these changes appear to be long-term, and may contribute to the development of diseases that have been linked to sleep deprivation in epidemiological research." (Vilma A, et al 2013)

Not only has the connection between lack of sleep and suppressed immunity been made, there has also been research that clearly shows a correlation between *interrupted* sleep and cancer growth.

In a study done in October 2013, researchers from the University of Chicago studied two groups of mice. One group was allowed to sleep peacefully while the second group had their sleep interrupted at regular intervals. This was continued for a period of one week before cancer cells were injected into both groups of mice.

Subsequent testing revealed that while both groups of mice developed tumors, the tumors of the mice whose sleep was interrupted had tumors that were *twice as large* and much more aggressive. (Hakim F, et al. 2014)

What the researchers found was that the mice that were allowed uninterrupted sleep had more immune cells known as TAMs or M1-type tumor-associated macrophages, whose function is to support the immune system and attack cancer cells.

However, the mice whose sleep had been interrupted had more of the immune cells known as M2-TAMs, which actually suppress the immune system and support tumor growth via blood vessels. In other words, they feed the tumors.

It's important to note that the mice with the aggressive tumors only had their sleep interrupted for one week prior to being injected with the cancer cells. It's clear that lack of sleep or sleep that is erratic or unrestful has a profound impact on our immune systems and does so in a very short time.

Improving Your Sleep Patterns to Protect Your Immune System
There are a number of factors that work against getting adequate and peaceful sleep.

Adults today are often struggling to keep up with extremely demanding schedules that force them to forgo sleep in exchange for getting (almost) everything done. Marriage, relationships, caring for children and aged parents, career and community involvement all seem to require first-place priority on our to-do lists.

Anxiousness due to work, finances and relationships often make it hard to fall asleep, leaving us lying awake at night with minds that refuse to be quieted.

A diet high in caffeine, sugar and starch also have a serious effect on how easily we can fall to sleep and how well we're able to stay asleep.

However, there are a number of things that we can do to keep lack of quality sleep from having a negative impact on our immune systems.

Make sleep the priority that it should be.
If you regularly and voluntarily sleep less than eight hours because your schedule is too demanding, reexamine your priorities.

Track how you're spending your mornings and evenings for a week or so and decide what can be exchanged for better health. Spend less time cleaning up at night and resolve to catch up on your days off. Turn off the TV mid-evening rather than staying up late to catch the late-night talk show. If you frequently bring home work, vow to put it aside by 8 or 9pm. Instead of getting up an hour early every morning, spend a few minutes in the evening laying out everyone's clothing for the next day as well as some ready-to-eat breakfast foods such as cereal, muffins and fruit. Then set your alarm for a later time in the morning.

Establish a sleep routine.

Parents of young children know that they go to sleep more easily if they have an established routine. The same is true of adults. A standard routine that lasts about thirty minutes before bed sends a signal to our brains that it's time for sleep.

You can have any routine you like, as long as it works for you. Warm showers or baths, a cup of herbal tea or reading in bed are all things you might include. The important thing is to have a routine and to do it at (at least roughly) the same time every night.

Studies have shown that this type of preparation helps us to fall asleep more quickly and easily.

Get a minimum of 7 hours sleep, every day.
Commit to getting between 7-8 hours of sleep
every day and to getting it at pretty much the
same time every day where you possibly can.
Even if you work at night and sleep during the
day, it's important to go to bed at the same time
every day, within an hour or so. Some studies
have shown that regularity of sleep is almost as
important as the quantity.

Get a handle on caffeine.
Almost everyone loves a great cup of coffee or
tea and there's no reason you shouldn't enjoy
yours. However, try to limit yourself to 2-3 cups
of caffeinated beverages per day and have your
last one at least five hours before bedtime.

Limit nighttime sugar and carbs.
Evening snacks are one of the simple pleasures
in life, especially with a great book or favorite
movie. However, snacks high in sugar and
simple carbs, such as desserts, breads and
cereals, should be off-limits within three hours of
bedtime.

If you're a person who loves a sweet treat in the
evening, have it right after dinner, rather than a

few hours later in front of the TV. If you're hungry close to bedtime, stick with protein and fat-rich foods such as cold meats, warm milk, nuts, seeds or some cheese. This will ensure that your blood sugar isn't sky high when you're trying to rest. Also, the Omega-3 fats and selenium in some of these foods reduce anxiety and promote sleep.

Limit alcohol in the evenings.
Many people think that a "nightcap" helps them to feel sleepy and get a better night's rest. However, that's not exactly true. While alcohol may help you to fall asleep, sleep studies have shown that drinking alcohol within a few hours of bed will actually result in more wakefulness during the night.

Cut off the electronics.
Several recent studies have shown that electronics interfere with our ability to sleep.

The artificial light from computer screens, televisions, tablets and even our phones lowers the amount of melatonin in our bloodstreams. Melatonin is a hormone that promotes calm, restfulness and sleep. Some studies indicate that melatonin levels drop by as much as 22%

after two hours of exposure to electronic screens.

Either limit your evening screen time to an hour or less or try to set a cut-off time for checking email, surfing the net, watching TV, and texting friends or playing games on your phone. That cutoff time should be at least two hours before you plan to go to bed.

By taking steps to get enough restful sleep, you'll not only boost your immune system, but have more energy, improved memory and mental focus and more stable moods.

Step Four: Boosting Your Immunity by Promoting a Healthy Liver

When most people think about liver health, they usually think of limiting alcohol intake. While excessive drinking can tax the liver, toxins present a serious danger to our immune systems by damaging liver function.

Our livers are charged with filtering out toxins before they reach our bloodstreams. However, environmental toxins, toxins and metals in our foods and an excess of free radicals all impair our liver's ability to do its job.

In addition to limiting exposure to these toxins, one of the most important things we can do to support liver function as part of our immune system is to eat foods that are high in an antioxidant called glutathione.

Glutathione is a combination of three important amino acids: cysteine, glutamine and glycine. Glutathione actually recycles the antioxidants in our bodies so that they can be used to their maximum disease-fighting potential. In fact, in studies on individual cells, glutathione has been shown to prevent some cancers.

(Scholz RW. Graham KS. Gumpricht E. Reddy CC. 1989: 570)

The power of glutathione is in its high sulfur content. Sulfur actually acts as a sticky surface to which toxins adhere. The sulfur then takes the toxins with it as it passes from the body in urine (Hyman 2010). Unfortunately, although our bodies do make some glutathione, it's not enough to compete with all of the toxins our bodies are subjected to on a daily basis.

Fortunately, we can easily boost glutathione levels in our bodies by eating foods that a rich in this micronutrient.

These include garlic and onions as well as all cruciferous vegetables such as cabbage, brussels sprouts, kale, collards and mustard greens. Whey protein is also a good source, but it must be biologically-active (unpasteurized) and denatured whey protein.

Step Five: Boosting Your Immunity by Improving Digestive Health

Your digestive system is responsible for ridding your body of the stored wastes and toxins that promote inflammation and hamper the immune system. Having a digestive system that is operating on a highly-functional level is essential to improving your body's ability to protect itself against diseases, including all forms of cancer.

The two best things you can do for digestive health are to get plenty of clean water and to eat a diet that is high in plant fibers (both soluble and insoluble) and low in processed foods.

119

We'll talk more about an immune-boosting diet in the next section, but for the purposes of the digestive system, plant fibers (as opposed to grain fibers) are like a whisk broom for the digestive tract. They help to clean away toxic buildup and the build-up of stored fats, gluten and wastes in the intestines.

Processed foods work against digestive health in a number of ways. Unhealthy fats and refined sugars and flours slow metabolism, upset the balance of digestive enzymes and provide very little of the fiber you need to carry these things back *out* of your body.

You also need a great deal of pure water on a daily basis, to help your digestive system to function regularly and optimally. Water is also needed to help your kidneys to work properly. The kidneys support the immune system by filtering out toxins and sending them out of the body in your urine.

Step Six: Boosting Your Immunity through Proper Diet

Proper diet supports healthy immune function more than perhaps any other step you can take.

We've already talked about how eliminating processed foods will reduce the number of harmful toxins in your system and promote digestive health. But there is so much more that the right diet can do to vastly improve your immunity.

Get plenty of plant foods in a wide variety.
Our bodies need a huge quantity and variety of antioxidants in order to fuel our immune systems. Unfortunately, very few people eat a diet that is rich enough in these antioxidants to make a difference.

Multivitamins are not necessarily the best answer. Many multivitamins are made with sub-standard ingredients, contain additives, binding agents and fillers and too few of the antioxidants we need.

Additionally, much of the micronutrient content in multivitamins is rendered useless by the acids in our stomachs before it can be metabolized and absorbed into our bloodstream. Whole foods are a much better and much more bio-available resource.

In particular, a variety of fresh plant foods should be an essential part of your daily diet.

Vegetables and fruits are loaded with antioxidants and phytonutrients that are known to boost the immune system.

The best way to ensure that you get a wide variety of these micronutrients is to get a wide variety of fruits and vegetables.

Fruits and vegetables in certain color groups tend to have the same antioxidants and phytonutrients. In other words, blue and purple produce has one set of antioxidants while orange or red plants have another.

Without getting into an exhaustive list of which group has which nutrients, if you eat at least some foods in each color group every day, you're quite likely to get all of the antioxidants you need.

Typically, the deeper or darker the color of the food, the more antioxidants it contains. Here are some of the best choices in each color group:

Red: Tomatoes, watermelon, red grapes, red apples, beets, Swiss chard and red berries.

Blue/Purple: Concord grapes, blueberries, blackberries, plums, eggplant.

Yellow/Orange: Summer squash, winter squash, sweet potatoes, oranges, grapefruit, carrots.

Green: Kiwi, kale, spinach, broccoli, Brussel sprouts, parsley, cucumber, Collard greens, mustard greens, Romaine lettuce.

Try to get at least one food from each group each day. We have a tendency to stick to just a few favorite fruits and vegetables, which limits the variety of antioxidants in our diet but also robs us of the pleasure of variety in flavor and texture.

Make a commitment to buy at least one new fruit or vegetable every week. It might be something you've never tried or just something you don't eat at home or eat very often. Visit farmer's markets to get inspired, get some great recipes and get some fun out of this healthy step.

Get plenty of Omega-3 fatty acids.
Omega-3 fatty acids get plenty of publicity for boosting heart health and improving mental and emotional health as well. However, they are also an important anti-inflammatory.

The best sources for omega-3 fats are flax seeds and walnuts, and wild-caught, cold-water fish such as salmon, sardines, haddock and cod. But grass-fed beef and game, pasture-raised eggs, shrimp, Brussels sprouts and cauliflower are also good sources.

You should note that grass-fed meats and poultry are high in Omega-3 fats while those raised in commercial feedlots are not, so please choose organic, grass-fed meats as much as is possible.

This brings us to our next point.

Eat organic as much as possible.
Continuing to eat fruits, vegetables, grains, dairy and meats that are loaded with pesticides, herbicides and hormones is counterproductive to everything else you're doing to boost your immunity. These are the very things that are already suppressing your immune system, so you need to limit them as much as you can.

Many people think they can't afford to eat a largely organic diet, but this isn't necessarily true. Yes, organic foods do cost more in the supermarket, but they're often available at a much lower cost in farmer's markets.

You can also free up more grocery money by eating less meat but making it organic, skipping the processed and packaged foods and using that money for organic dairy and produce and cutting out a couple of restaurant meals or several gourmet coffees each month and adding the money to your grocery budget. Affording organic and grass-fed foods isn't really that difficult, it just requires some new and creative thinking.

Be sensitive to your sensitivities.
While food sensitivities aren't as dangerous as food allergies, many people underestimate the toll they can take on the immune system. If dairy, sugar, flour or gluten make you feel bloated, gassy, fatigued or otherwise uncomfortable, you need to strictly limit them.

Many people love their ice cream or yeast rolls to the extent that they're willing to put up with the mild discomfort later, but your immune system sees these foods as invaders and is working to protect you from them. This just overburdens your immune system and uses up resources that would be better spent elsewhere. If you suspect that you might have an actual food allergy such as lactose-intolerance or

Celiac disease, by all means get tested and if so, eliminate them from your diet.

If you're just a bit sensitive to these foods and don't want to cut them from your diet, at least try to make them very special treats to be enjoyed very rarely.

A good way to find out if you might be sensitive to a certain food (and it's difficult to tell if you have a poor diet all around) is to stop eating it for two weeks. Note how you feel at the end of this time, including your energy level, whether you feel less bloated and if you have more regular elimination. Then add the food back in. If you're sensitive to it, you'll probably notice a change in how you feel within just a few days. Then it's up to you to decide if that food is really worth the problems it's causing.

Eliminate or severely limit processed foods.
Processed, pre-made, packaged and fast foods are loaded with pesticides, herbicides, hormones, antibiotics, artificial sweeteners, sugar and hydrogenated fats.

Try to make whole, fresh foods 90% or more of your daily diet. While you can't be expected to do without all packaged foods, right down to your condiments, you should strive to eliminate as many of them as possible.

Particularly bad are packaged snacks like chips, cookies, cakes, cereals and other baked goods. This doesn't mean you have to do without them entirely. Homemade versions are much better for you, as you control the ingredients. If you have a weight problem, limiting your treats to homemade varieties will help you to limit calories as well, since you're likely to choose a piece of fruit or some nuts instead of pulling out your mixer.

Boosting your immune system through choosing a more nutritious diet shouldn't be seen as a chore or a deprivation. Most people find that once they adjust to eating more whole foods and fewer processed foods, they learn to enjoy a wider variety of food and get more pleasure from their meals.

Eating to boost your immune system doesn't mean going without your favorite "junk" foods or treats forever. By all means, enjoy a great slice of pizza or your favorite candy bar every now and then, but consider it a well-deserved reward for eating healthily the other 90% of the time. Then you can savor it without feeling guilty and without harming your health.

Step Seven: Boosting Your Immunity through Exercise

We all know that exercise helps us to maintain a healthy weight, build and preserve muscle tissue, improve heart health and build strong bones. However, several studies have shown that exercise also helps to boost our immune systems. Although the reasons for this are still up for debate, there are several predominant theories:

- Physical activity may help by flushing bacteria out from the lungs (thus decreasing the chance of a cold, flu, or other airborne illness) and may flush out cancer-causing cells (carcinogens) by increasing output of wastes, such as urine and sweat.

- Exercise sends antibodies and white blood cells (the body's defense cells) through the body at a quicker rate. As these antibodies or white blood cells circulate more rapidly, they could detect illnesses earlier than they might normally. The increased rate of circulating blood may also trigger the release of hormones that "warn" immune cells of intruding bacteria or viruses.

- The temporary rise in body temperature may prevent bacterial growth, allowing the body to fight the infection more effectively. (This is similar to what happens when the body has a fever.)

- Exercise slows down the release of stress-related hormones. Stress increases the chance of illness.

    (National Library of Medicine Reviewed 2012)

Even if you are not a fan of working out, you can still get enough exercise to support a robust immune system. Even thirty minutes of moderate walking, swimming or cycling, three times per week, has been shown to have a positive effect on immunity.

If you don't care for walking, swimming or cycling, try taking a dance class, having fun with a Zumba DVD at home, playing outdoors with the kids or playing a regular game of tennis, basketball or soccer. Anything that gets you moving at a moderate pace for 20-30 minutes will do.

Conclusion

Finding out that you have a potentially cancerous condition is never an easy thing.

Initially, emotions run high and they run the gamut from anger to fear to sadness and indignation. We *don't* want to know that we're at a higher risk of cancer. We *don't* want to change our lifestyle or habits and we *don't* want to be constantly worrying and watching.

Those are all natural reactions. Processing your diagnosis and what it means to your life is a lot like going through the steps of the grieving process.

But, a diagnosis of actinic keratosis is not a death sentence, nor is it a guarantee that you'll have to do battle with squamous cell carcinoma at some point in your future.

However, it is an alert that you are to some extent predisposed to squamous cell carcinoma and that you do need to be careful and to make any changes to your lifestyle necessary to prevent additional lesions and catch any new lesions as early as possible.

It's important, though, to maintain a positive attitude toward your diagnosis and toward living with actinic keratosis. A positive attitude reduces stress, which has been definitively linked to cancer growth. A positive attitude also allows you to get on with enjoying your life.

After all, you got a diagnosis of actinic keratosis, not cancer. The fact is that a warning such as this can be a wonderful catalyst for positive change.

People who have survived various types of cancer often report that their lives are fuller, richer and more fulfilling after cancer than they were before. They're keenly aware that they've been given a second chance to take better care of themselves, make healthier choices and to do the things they always meant to do "later," the things they regretted not doing when they were first diagnosed.

Finding out that you have a "precancerous" condition can stimulate those kinds of positive change as well. *You* have a chance to create a healthier lifestyle. *You* have a chance to do things you've been putting off. *You* have a new motivation to take more chances, live more intentionally and pay attention to what really matters to you.

Focusing on those things will not only help you to stay healthy, but to appreciate that health as fully and actively as you possibly can.

Glossary of Terms

Actinic keratosis: A benign lesion on or just below the skin's surface that is caused by sun damage. Actinic keratosis can lead to squamous cell carcinoma.

Bowen's disease: The earliest stage of squamous cell carcinoma. Also known as Bowenoid actinic keratosis or in situ squamous cell carcinoma.

Chemical peel therapy: The use of Jessner's solution or trichloroacetic acid (TCA) to remove actinic keratoses. Considered a non-invasive form of removal.

Cryotherapy: The use of nitrogen to freeze and kill an actinic keratosis lesion.

Curettage: Removal of a lesion using a small scalpel or curette.

Diclofenac: Topical cream often used in conjunction with other forms of treatment, typically on patients who are not suited for other types of therapy.

Dysplastic nevi: Benign and very common skin lesions that are often mistaken (by laypersons) for skin cancer or actinic keratosis.

Fluorouracil 5%: A form of chemotherapy available in a cream and applied to the skin. Also known as 5-FU, Carac, Fluoroplex, Efudex and 5-Fluorouracil.

Imiquimod: Also known as Aldara, Zyclara, and Beseina. Topical cream which stimulates the immune response and helps the body to manufacture interferon.

Ingenol mebutate: Sold under the brand name Picato, this is a newly approved (2012) topical gel whose results have not yet been fully documented.

Laser therapy or removal: The use of an erbium YAG or carbon dioxide laser to remove an actinic keratosis lesion without causing bleeding or more than minor pain.

Photodynamic therapy: Also referred to as blue light therapy, phototherapy and photodynamic therapy. Application of a chemical such as Levulan or Kerastick to a lesion and then exposing it to powerful light.

Squamous cell carcinoma: One of three types of skin cancer. Squamous cell carcinoma is one

of the easiest skin cancers to treat when caught
in its early stages.

Resources

The following is a list of websites and organizations that you may find very helpful in learning about and living with actinic keratosis.

Skin Cancer Foundation – An excellent US research site with explanations of treatment options and statistics as well as images of actinic keratoses.
http://www.skincancer.org/skin-cancer-information/actinic-keratosis

Patient.co.uk – Very good UK site with detailed information and excellent images for actinic keratosis.
http://www.patient.co.uk/doctor/Actinic-(Solar)-Keratosis.htm

Primary Care Dermatology Society – Excellent UK site primarily aimed at medical professionals, but with a large collection of actinic keratoses images.
http://www.pcds.org.uk/clinical-guidance/actinic-keratosis-syn.-solar-keratosis#images

National Center for Biotechnology Information: A service of the US National Library of Medical Science, National Institutes of

Health. Excellent information on treatment, risk factors and prognosis statistics.
http://www.ncbi.nlm.nih.gov/pubmedhealth/PMH0001830/

Medicine Net – Very good US site geared toward patients rather than the medical community. Good information that is easy to understand.
http://www.medicinenet.com/actinic_keratosis/article.htm#what_is_an_actinic_keratosis_and_what_does_it_look_like

Works Cited

"A Report of the Surgeon General: How Tobacco Smoke Causes Disease -The Biology and Behavioral Basis for Smoking-Attributable Disease." *SurgeonGeneral.gov.* 2014. http://www.surgeongeneral.gov/library/reports/tobaccosmoke/factsheet.html (accessed January 25, 2014).

Actinic keratosis. November 2011. http://www.pcds.org.uk/clinical-guidance/actinic-keratosis-syn.-solar-keratosis (accessed January 1, 2014).

Actinic Keratosis. 2013. http://www.skincancer.org/skin-cancer-information/actinic-keratosis (accessed January 2, 2014).

American Cancer Society. *Cancer.org.* 2013. http://www.cancer.org/treatment/treatmentsandsideeffects/guidetocancerdrugs/imiquimod-cream (accessed January 14, 2014).

American Psychological Association. *Stress Weakens the Immune System*. n.d. http://www.apa.org/research/action/immune.aspx (accessed January 24, 2014).

Cole MD, Gary. "Actinic Keratosis." *MedicineNet.com.* August 2013. http://www.medicinenet.com/actinic_keratosis/article.htm (accessed January 12, 2014).

E.Miller, Susan C Segerstrom and Gregory. " Psychological Stress and the Human Immune System." *National Library of Medicine (National Institutes of Health).* n.d. http://www.ncbi.nlm.nih.gov/pmc/articles/PMC1361287/ (accessed January 14, 2014).

Habif, TP. "Principles of diagnosis and anatomy." In *Clinical Dermatology, 5th edition*, Capter 1. St. Louis, MO: Mosby Elsevier, 2009.

Hakim F, et al. "Fragmented sleep accelerates tumor growth and progression through recruitment of tumor-associated

macrophages and TLR4 signaling."
Journal of Cancer Research, 2014.

Hyman, Mark. "Essential Glutathione - The
Mother of All Antioxidants." *Dr. Mark
Hyman.* May 19, 2010.
http://drhyman.com/blog/2010/05/19/glut
athione-the-mother-of-all-antioxidants/
(accessed January 25, 2014).

James C, Crawford R, Martika M. Actinic
Keratosis. In: C. James, R. Crawford, M.
Martinka, and R. Marks. "Skin Tumors."
In *WHO Pathology and Genetics*, 30-33.
Lyon: IARC Press, 2006.

Kour K, Pandey A, Suri KA, Satti NK, Gupta KK,
Bani S. "Restoration of stress-induced
altered T cell function and corresponding
cytokines patterns by Withanolide A. ."
*Int Immunopharmacol. 2009
Sep;9(10):1137-44.*, 2009 :
Sep;9(10):1137-44.

Lawrence N, Cox SE, Cockerell CJ, Freeman
RG, Cruz PD Jr. "A comparison of the
efficacy and safety of Jessner's solution
and 35% trichloroacetic acid vs 5%

fluorouracil in the treatment of
widespread facial actinic keratoses."
Archives of Dermatology, 1995: 176-81.

Love WE, et al. "Topical imiquimod or
fluorouracil therapy for basal and
squamous cell carcinoma: A systematic
review." *Archives of Dermatology*, 2009:
145(12): 1431-1438.

Lubritz RR, Smolewski SA. "Cryosurgery cure
rate of actinic keratoses." *Journal of
American Academy of Dermatology*,
1982: 631-2.

Marks R; Rennie G; Selwood TS. "Malignant
transformation of solar keratoses to
squamous cell carcinoma." *Lancet*, 1988:
795-7.

Mayo Clinic Staff. *Squamous cell carcinoma.*
n.d. http://www.mayoclinic.org/diseases-
conditions/squamous-cell-
carcinoma/basics/definition/con-
20037813 (accessed January 24, 2014).

MF, Holick. "Vitamin D and Health: Evolution,
Biologic Functions, and Recommended
Dietary Intakes of Vitamin D." In *Vitamin*

D: Physiology, Molecular Biology and Clinical Applications , by Holick MF. Humana Press, 2010.

National Library of Medicine, National Institutes of Health. "Exercise and Immunity." *Medline Plus Medical Encyclopedia.* May 18, Reviewed 2012. http://www.nlm.nih.gov/medlineplus/ency/article/007165.htm (accessed January 23, 2014).

RG, Glogau. "The risk of progression to invasive disease." *Journal of American Academy of Dermatology (42)*, 2000: 23-4.

Rigel DS, Stein Gold LF. "The importance of early diagnosis and treatment of actinic keratosis." *Journal of the American Academy of Dermotology*, 2013.

Scholz RW. Graham KS. Gumpricht E. Reddy CC. . "Mechanism of interaction of vitamin E and glutathione in the protection against membrane lipid peroxidation." *Annals of the New York Academy of Science 1989:570:514-7.* , 1989: 570: 514-7.

Skin Cancer Foundation. *squamous cell carcinoma treatment options.* n.d. (accessed January 24, 2014).

—. *Suamous Cell Carcinoma Causes and Risk Factors.* n.d. http://www.skincancer.org/skin-cancer-information/squamous-cell-carcinoma/scc-causes-and-risk-factors (accessed January 24, 2014).

Sopori, M. "Effects of cigarette smoke on the immune system." *Nature Journal - Immunology University of California at Berkeley,* 2002.

"Squamous Cell Carcinoma." *skincancer.org.* n.d. http://www.skincancer.org/skin-cancer-information/squamous-cell-carcinoma (accessed January 24, 2014).

Thai KE, Fergin P, Freeman M, Vinciullo C, Francis D, Spelman L, et al. "A prospective study of the use of cryosurgery for the treatment of actinic keratoses." *International Journal of Dermatology,* 2004: 687-92.

Turner EH, Loftis JM, Blackwell AD. "Serotonin a la carte: supplementation with the serotonin precursor 5-hydroxytryptophan." *Pharmacological Therapy*, 2006: 109 (3): 325–38.

Unknown. "Stress Weakens the Immune System n.d." *American Psychological Association.* n.d. http://www.apa.org/research/action/immune.aspx (accessed January 24, 2014).

US National Library of Medicine and National Institutes of Health. *Squamous cell carcinoma.* n.d. http://www.nlm.nih.gov/medlineplus/ency/article/000829.htm (accessed January 24, 2014).

Vilma A, et al. "Partial Sleep Restriction Activates Immune Response-Related Gene Expression Pathways: Experimental and Epidemiological Studies in Humans." *PLoS ONE*, 2013.

Wood B, Rea MS, Plitnick B, Figueiro MG. "Light level and duration of exposure determine the impact of self-luminous

tablets on melatonin suppression."
Applied Ergonomics, 2013: 44(2);237-40.

CPSIA information can be obtained
at www.ICGtesting.com
Printed in the USA
BVHW041405281019
562265BV00012B/754/P

9 780992 798550